Vest Pocket Fat Counter

Susan Kagen Podell, M.S., R.D.

Doubleday
New York London Toronto Sydney Auckland

PUBLISHED BY DOUBLEDAY
a division of Bantam Doubleday Dell Publishing Group, Inc.
666 Fifth Avenue, New York, New York 10103

DOUBLEDAY and the portrayal of an anchor with a dolphin
are trademarks of Doubleday,
a division of Bantam Doubleday Dell Publishing Group, Inc.

Library of Congress Cataloging-in-Publication Data
Podell, Susan Kagen.
    Vest pocket fat counter / Susan Kagen Podell.—1st ed.
        p.   cm.
    Includes bibliographical references.
    1. Food—Fat content—Tables.   I. Title.
TX553.L5P64   1992
641.1'4—dc20   91-33022
                                                   CIP

ISBN 0-385-42294-6
Copyright © 1992 by Susan Kagen Podell, M.S., R.D.

Contents

Introduction

Fat ... It's become the hottest topic and biggest concern on the American nutrition agenda. But what is a gram of fat and how many do you need? What is the impact of various fats on your blood cholesterol level? How does "life in the fat lane" affect your weight? What are the cancer risks associated with high fat intake? This little book is the key to understanding the whole fat story: from fat grams to fake fats. So read on and learn what the health authorities already know ... that Americans eat too much fat and the way to trim inches and boost heart health is to slash the fat!

Why Lower Fat?
Government Guidelines

The Surgeon General of the United States, in one of the most extensive reports to date on nutrition, identified FAT—not sodium, not cholesterol, and not preservatives or pesticides—as the top dietary priority for this country. In fact, it was noted that five of the leading causes of death in the United States are linked to a fatty diet. The new 1990 *Dietary Guidelines for Americans*, published every five years by the federal government, recommended that Americans "choose a diet low in fat . ." It goes on to say that populations like ours, with diets high in fat, have more obesity, cancer, diabetes, and heart disease than populations who eat less fat. Our diets are literally making us sick!

Facts on Fats—Total Fat Budget

All fat is fattening! Fat has over twice as many calories as carbohydrates or protein. Americans tend to eat about 40% of their calories from fat. As a country, we are bursting at the seams! You should get no more than 30% (or less than one third) of your calories from fat. But how do you go about figuring what is 30%? Bring a calculator to the table? Take all the food you eat and discard one third? Avoid ALL fatty foods? Of course not. The following is a simple plan for **budgeting** your fat intake. The upper limit for the fat grams in your diet depends on the calories you eat. To make sure that no more than 30% of your calories come from fat, you must first decide how many calories you want to eat and then use this simple chart as a guide . . . But, forget about counting calories, count fat grams instead!! The real bonus of counting fat grams is that once you have reached your daily limit, there are still plenty of delicious, virtually fat-free foods you can still eat!!

Calories	Fat grams
1000	30
1200	40
1500	50
1800	60
2000	67
2200	73
2500	83
2800	93
3000	100

Remember, these numbers represent UPPER LIMITS for fat intake. *Less is better!*

But just what is a gram of fat? A gram is a unit of weight like ounces or pounds. It weighs about as much as a paper clip. There are 28 grams in an ounce. Each gram of fat contains 9 calories, as opposed to 4 calories for the same weight of carbohydrate or protein. Thus, fat has more than twice as many calories, gram for gram, as carbohydrate or protein. Fat is fattening because a small amount is loaded with calories. **Just by limiting your fat grams, you'll automatically be cutting your calories!**

Fat grams are generally given per serving of food. Unfortunately, most people underestimate the size of their servings. Learning to measure accurately is essential to limiting your fat. Three ounces of meat, for example, is considered a "standard size." That's about the size of a deck of cards. Many people eat much more. Depending on the food, servings may be listed by the teaspoon, tablespoon, cup, or ounce. It's helpful to weigh and measure food from time to time to get a realistic picture of the quantity of food you eat. The final challenge is to juggle all foods eaten in a day so that they add up to no more than your budgeted fat allowance.

For those of you who are math buffs, the following arithmetic will determine the percentage of calories in food that come from fat:

1. multiply the number of grams of fat in food by 9.
2. multiply the answer in step one by 100.
3. divide the answer of step two by the total number of calories in a serving of the food. This number should be no more than 30.

The following two food label examples will help explain this concept better.

| *Budget Gourmet* vs. | *Healthy Choice* |
| Chicken Au Gratin | Sirloin Beef Tips |

Nutritional Information Per Serving

Serving size: 9.1 oz	Serving size: 11.75 oz
Servings per container: 1	Servings per container: 1
Calories: 260	Calories: 290
Protein: 20 g	Protein: 25 g
Carbohydrate: 21 g	Carbohydrate: 33 g
Fat: 11 g	**Fat: 6 g**

11 g fat × 9 cal/g	6 g fat × 9 cal/g
= 99 cal as fat	= 54 cal as fat
99 × 100 = 9900	54 × 100 = 5400
9900 ÷ 260 total	5400 ÷ 290 total
calories = 38%	calories = 19%
calories as fat	calories as fat

Healthy Choice Beef Sirloin Tips is a lean choice, while *Budget Gourmet* Chicken Au Gratin is a high fat choice. In other words, the lower-fat dinner can provide a 23% larger portion, while only adding a mere 30 extra calories.

A single food may contain more than 30% of calories from fat, however, and still fit into a healthy eating plan that has no more than 30% of the total day's calories from fat. For example, a low-calorie margarine with only 5 grams of fat per tablespoon gets 90%–100% of its calories from fat. It would be misleading to suggest that this is not a smart food choice. Remember, it's all in how you budget your fat for the day. So, forget percentages and focus on grams!

Be careful of foods that are promoted as being low in fat, however. Misleading claims usually mean that the product has a low percentage of fat *by weight*, not a low percentage *of calories* as fat. For example, hot dogs are only about 30% fat by weight, but are almost 93% calories as fat. In other words, when a food is labeled "70% fat free," it really means that 30% of the product weight is FAT, but 93% of the calories come from FAT!! Remember to check the label for the fat grams and to count them in your budget.

The recommended shift to a low-fat diet has one more catch. Fats in foods are mixtures of saturated and unsaturated fat. While you want to reduce ALL fat you eat to under 30% of calories, you must limit saturated fats more than unsaturated fats. Saturated fat raises blood cholesterol levels, while unsaturated fats do not.

Saturated Fat:
The Artery Clogger

Much like dietary cholesterol, saturated fats are mostly found in animal products—mainly red meats, whole milk, cream, cheese, butter, lard, and chicken skin. Unlike dietary cholesterol, however, saturated fat is also found in certain vegetable sources—coconut oil, palm oil, and cocoa butter. These vegetable fats are known as the tropical oils and are generally found in store-bought baked products and chocolate. All saturated fats tend to be hard at room temperature, such as the fat on a steak or a stick of butter. Another form of saturated fat is *hydrogenated* fat. By a chemical process, food manufacturers change liquid vegetable oils into solid fats. As the liquid hardens, the amount of saturated fat increases. The best example of this process is a stick margarine versus a tub margarine. Since the stick is harder, it is more saturated than tub margarine. Crisco 100% vegetable shortening, which is quite solid at room temperature, is also a highly hydrogenated or saturated fat. Read labels on all foods to determine if hydrogenated (or partially hydrogenated) fat has been used in the processing.

Unsaturated Fat: Heart Smart

There are two types of unsaturated fat: **polyunsaturated** and **monounsaturated**. Polyunsaturated fats are oils from a variety of plant products. Corn, safflower, sunflower, and soybean oils are all highly polyunsaturated. All polyunsaturated fats are liquid at room temperature. These fats lower blood cholesterol levels—both the "bad" LDL's and the "good" HDL's. (LDL's—low density lipoproteins—are responsible for most of the plaque buildup in the arteries. HDL's—high density lipoproteins—are responsible for carrying cholesterol away from the heart to the liver, where it can be removed from the blood.) Years ago, doctors and nutritionists were recommending that patients with high blood cholesterol counts drink small amounts of corn oil to help lower their cholesterol. However, in an effort to keep TOTAL FAT low and avoid reducing "good" HDL's too much, this practice is no longer prescribed. In addition, recent research has implicated polyunsaturated fats in the development of breast cancer. Another category of polyunsaturated fats is the Omega-3 fatty acids found in cold-water marine animals, especially fish. Although these fish oils have received much media attention in recent years, research is inconclusive regarding their effect on blood cholesterol or other blood components. Therefore, while fish itself is a delicious, low-fat meal, it would be unwise for you to try fish oil pills without the advice of your doctor or registered dietitian.

Monounsaturated fats are also fats of plant origin. Sources include olive oil and olives, canola oil, sesame oil and seeds, peanut oil and peanuts, almonds, walnuts, and avocados. Until several years ago, monounsaturated fats were considered neutral, that is, having no effect on blood cholesterol levels. Recent research, however, indicates that monounsaturated fats, like polyunsaturated fats, lower blood cholesterol levels, but this reduction affects primarily the "bad" LDL's. It has little effect on the "good" HDL's. In other words, monounsaturated fat does not rid the body of the helpful, "good" HDL's. Research indicates that these fats are the "*safest*" of all, having little negative association with heart disease or cancer. One third to one half of the total fat in your diet, therefore, should come from monounsaturated fats. Be careful when choosing peanut butter, however. Although peanut oil is monounsaturated, most national brands of peanut butter contain lots of hydrogenated (saturated) fat. Try a natural peanut butter instead.

The Fat Loading Duo:
• Lipoprotein Lipase and Yo-Yo Dieting •

Fat's tendency to stick to the ribs (and hips and stomach) seems to be dependent, at least partially, on your previous dieting habits. It seems that lipoprotein lipase or LPL, an enzyme responsible for loading fat into fat cells, acts differently in yo-yo dieters than in those who have never been overweight. When previously overweight people eat fat, their LPL levels rise above normal, thus allowing them to *store more fat*. They literally become extra efficient at storing dietary fat as body fat. Dieting rules used to say that if you ate a 1200-calorie-per-day diet, regardless of whether the calories came from carbohydrate, protein, or fat, you'd lose weight. We now know that just isn't true. Fat calories get metabolized differently than carbohydrate or protein calories and they come perfectly shaped for storage. In other words, your body doesn't have to burn any calories to convert fat to a storable form (as it does for carbohydrate and protein calories). Clearly, fat calories are particularly good at making fat bodies!! They are just more fattening!!

•   **Fake Fats**   •

If you've been thinking that you'll never be able to eat ice cream or french fries again—read on. The new fat substitutes, Simplesse and Olestra, have emerged out of our new awareness of the excess fat in our diets and our desire to still eat delicious, creamy, fatty foods!

Simplesse was developed by the NutraSweet Company. It is made mainly from milk or egg protein and is being used in fat-free frozen ice cream, mayonnaise, cheese spread, and other fat-based dairy products. Simplesse was introduced in the new frozen dessert *Simple Pleasures*, which contains 120 calories and 1 g fat per 4-oz serving. Compared to traditional ice cream, which has 250 calories and 15 g fat per 4-oz serving, this is quite a fat bargain! Simplesse, however, is unsuitable for cooking or frying because it will congeal when heated. Simplesse is considered safe by all major government and consumer groups.

Olestra is the fat substitute developed by Procter & Gamble. It adds no calories or fats to products and can be used in cooking. French fries made in Olestra would shrink the calories per serving from 222 calories to 147 calories and would cut fat from 9 g to 2 g. Nevertheless, Olestra hasn't yet been approved by the FDA. Consumer groups are urging the government not to approve it until all safety questions have been resolved.

In the future, fat substitutes may allow us all to enjoy fatty foods with less guilt. But remember, they are not a panacea. The products containing these "fake fats" should be used in addition to a balanced low-fat diet.

Ten Fat-Free Alternatives

The following is a list of fat-free sauces and seasonings. Choose them to substitute for commonly used fatty ingredients.

1. Lemon juice.
2. Mustard.
3. Salsa or picante sauce.
4. Any specialty vinegar such as balsamic, tarragon, rosemary, or raspberry.
5. Bottled fat-free salad dressings or mayonnaise.
6. Bouillon, broth, or chilled and skimmed pan drippings. You can thicken any of these with flour or cornstarch for a fat-free gravy.
7. Plain fat-free yogurt.
8. Wine. When used in cooking, most alcohol calories will burn off, leaving only flavor.
9. Jams, jellies, or fruit spreads.
10. All herbs and spices.

Ten Easy Ways to Slash Fat from Your Diet

1. Choose skinless poultry, fish or shellfish, and lean cuts of red meat such as fillet, flank, rump, round, sirloin, or tenderloin. Avoid processed meats such as bacon, sausage, cold cuts, and all fat-marbled meats.
2. If you must fry food, use a non-stick pan with a cooking spray rather than adding oil.
3. Broil, bake, or grill meats on a rack so that the fat drips away.
4. Sauté foods in water and broth instead of oil or margarine.
5. Choose a low-fat margarine and fat-free mayonnaise or salad dressing.
6. Stretch fat-containing meats in recipes by thinly slicing and mixing with other ingredients such as vegetables and grains.
7. Substitute skim or 1% milk for 2% or whole milk at the table and in recipes.
8. Season foods with herbs and spices instead of margarine or butter.
9. Use skim milk cheese or other reduced-fat cheeses (with 5 g or less of fat per oz).
10. Cut the fat/oil in recipes by one third to one half, especially in recipes for quick breads or muffins, and casseroles or mixed dishes.

Ten Smart Snacking Tips

Choose	Instead of	Save
1 bagel	doughnut	16 g fat
2 Fig Newtons	2 brownies	10 g fat
1 oz pretzels	1 oz chips	8 g fat
1 C low-fat frozen yogurt	1 C Haagen-Däzs ice cream	16 g fat
10 jelly beans	2 Reese's peanut butter cups	11 g fat
1 C popcorn (unbuttered)	1 oz peanuts	13 g fat
28 gumdrops	1.59-oz pkg m & m's	10 g fat
1.5-oz pkg Good & Plenty	6 chocolate kisses	9 g fat
1 C seedless grapes	1 slice American cheese	9 g fat
15 Animal Crackers	3 oatmeal cookies	6 g fat

How to Use the Dial

The dial on the cover was designed to help you easily keep track of the fat in your diet. Remember your total fat limit for the day depends on the number of calories you need in a day. Use the fat gram budget provided at the beginning of the book to help you decide on your personal fat gram limit. Suppose for breakfast you wanted coffee with light cream and sugar, orange juice, corn flakes with one-half cup of whole milk, and two slices of toast with two pats of margarine. You would look up each food on the following food list, and move the dial the correct amount for each food. For example, since coffee, sugar, corn flakes, and orange juice contain virtually no fat, you would not move the dial at all. The toast contains about 2 g fat, the light cream contains another 3 g, the one-half cup whole milk contains 4.5 g, and the two pats margarine contain about 8 g fat for a total of 17.5 g fat at breakfast. If your fat gram limit for the day is say 40 g, you've already used up almost half of your daily fat and you've still got two meals to go, not to mention any snacks you might like! The importance of counting your fat grams is clear. The dial reminds you when to stop, go, or be cautious with certain foods and provides a simple method for keeping track of the fat in your diet.

Abbreviations

C	cup
env	envelope
fl	fluid
g	gram
lb	pound
lg	large
med	medium
oz	ounce
sm	small
sq	square
Tbsp	tablespoon
tsp	teaspoon
tr	trace
	(less than 1 g)
+	plus
pkg	package
pkt	packet

Weights and Measures

3 tsp = 1 Tbsp
2 Tbsp = 1 fl oz
4 Tbsp = $\frac{1}{4}$ C
8 Tbsp = $\frac{1}{2}$ C
16 Tbsp = 1 C or 8 fl oz
2 C = 16 fl oz or 1 lb

Food List

Note: *All information contained in this book is based on government sources or manufacturer labels and is listed in common household measures. Information is unavailable for some food products. For the most accurate, up-to-date information, make sure you become a label reader.*

BEVERAGES

		g Fat
Chocolate milk		
Whole	1 C (3.5% fat)	9
Low-fat	1 C (2% fat)	5
Low-fat	1 C (1% fat)	2.5
Coffee, black, instant or drip	1 Tbsp	tr
Coffee w/ 2 Tbsp light cream	1 C	6
Coffee, specialty, General Foods International	6 fl oz	2–3
Eggnog	1 C	16
Fruit juice (fresh or frozen, all varieties)	1 C	tr
Goat milk	1 C	10
Hot cocoa, Swiss Miss	1 env	3
Malted chocolate beverage whole milk + 3 tsp powder	1 C	10

		g Fat
Milk		
Whole	1 C (3.7 % fat)	9
Low-fat	1 C (2% fat)	5
Low-fat	1 C (1% fat)	3
Skim	1 C	tr
Buttermilk, cultured	1 C	2
Condensed, sweetened	1 C	27
Evaporated, canned	1 fl oz	2
Soft drinks, all varieties and brands	12 fl oz	tr
Tea, all varieties, regular or herbal	1 C	0
Vegetable juice, canned	6 fl oz	0

BREADSTUFF AND GRAINS

		g Fat
Breads		
Bagel, frozen		
Lender's, all varieties	1 each	1
Sara Lee, plain, onion, poppyseed, egg, cinnamon-raisin	1 each	2
Bran, honey	1 slice	1
French	1 slice	1
Italian	1 slice	1
Multigrain	1 slice	1
Oat	1 slice	2
Pita	1 piece	1

20

		g Fat
Pumpernickel	1 slice	1
Raisin	1 slice	1.5
Raisin-nut	1 slice	3
Rye	1 slice	1
Sourdough	1 slice	tr
White	1 slice	1
Whole wheat	1 slice	1
Croissant	1 each	9
English muffin	1 each	2

Muffin (from mix)

blueberry	1 each	7–8
banana-nut	1 each	7
bran	1 each	7
chocolate chip	1 each	8
corn	1 each	7

Crackers

Butter flavor

Ritz	4	4
Hi-Ho	4	5
Town House	5	5
Escort	3	4

Cheese

Nips	13	3
Cheez-It	12	4
Better Cheddar	11	4

Goldfish, Pepperidge
Farm Cheddar or

Parmesan	45	6

Matzo

egg	1 sq	2
plain	1 sq	tr

		g Fat
whole wheat	1 sq	1
Melba toast		
bacon or cheese	5	2
garlic, onion, rye, whole grain	5	1
pumpernickel or plain	3	0
sesame	5	2
Oysterettes	18	1
Peanut butter sandwich, toasted		
Keebler	1 pkg	9
Handi-snacks, with cheese	1 pkg	13
Scandinavian crispbreads		
Ideal, Kavli	2	0–tr
Wasa	1	0–1.5
Saltines, all brands	5	1–2
Soda or water, all brands	4	1
Wheat		
Keebler Harvest	3	4
Wheatsworth	5	3
Wheat Thins, plain	8	3
nutty	7	5
Triscuit	3	2
Sociables	6	3
Waffles, frozen		
Eggo regular, nutri-grain, or blueberry	1 each	5
bran	1 each	8
Roman Meal	1 each	7

		g Fat
Pancakes, frozen	3 med	3–6
Breakfast cereals		
All Bran/Bran Buds	1/3 C	tr
Alpha-bits	1 C	tr
Apple Jacks	1 C	tr
Bran, 100% or buds	1/2 C	tr
Bran Flakes, Kellogg's or Post	3/4 C	tr
Cap'n Crunch	3/4 C	tr
Cheerios	1 1/4 C	2
Chex, corn, rice, wheat	1 C	tr
Cocoa Puffs	1 C	1
Corn Flakes	1 C	tr
Cracklin' Oat Bran	1/3 C	4
Fruit Loops	1 C	tr
Fruit & Fibre	1/2 C	tr
Golden Grahams	3/4 C	1
Granola	1/3 C	6
Grape-nuts	1/4 C	tr
Kix	1 1/2 C	tr
Nutri-grain	3/4 C	tr
Product 19	3/4 C	tr
Puffed Rice or Wheat	1 C	tr
Quaker 100% Natural	1/4 C	6
Raisin Bran	3/4 C	tr
Rice Krispies	1 C	tr
Shredded Wheat	1 biscuit	tr
Special K	1 1/3 C	tr
Total	1 C	tr
Wheaties	1 C	tr

		g Fat
Rice, brown or white ... ½ C		tr
Rice products		
Long grain and wild rice from instant Minute Rice ½ C		4
Beef-flavored rice from instant Minute Rice ½ C		4
Chicken-flavored rice from instant Minute Rice ½ C		4
Chinese fried rice from instant Minute Rice ½ C		5
Spanich rice from instant Minute Rice ½ C		4
Frozen rice dishes, all brands ⅖ C		0–4
Pasta		
Noodles ⅗ C		1
chow mein ½ C		9
Ramen, all flavors 1 C		7–8
Romanoff, from mix ½ C		12
Stroganoff, from mix ½ C		12
Macaroni ⅗ C		tr
and cheese, mix, Kraft ¾ C		13
and cheese, canned, Franco-American ... $7\frac{3}{8}$ oz		5.5
and cheese, frozen, Banquet 8 oz		16

and beef, canned, Heinz	$7\frac{1}{4}$ oz	8
Spaghetti	1 C	tr
Spaghetti-O's	1 C	2
Spaghetti with tomato sauce and cheese, canned	1 C	2
Spaghetti with meat sauce, canned, Franco-American	1 C	10
Heinz	1 C	6
Spaghetti with tomato sauce and franks, canned	1 C	7
Spaghetti with tomato sauce, frozen		
Banquet	8 oz	15
Stouffer's	14 oz	12

DAIRY PRODUCTS

g Fat

Cheese		
American	1 oz	9
Blue	1 oz	8
Brick	1 oz	8
Brie	1 oz	8
Camembert	1 oz	7
Cheddar	1 oz	9
Cheese food, processed	1 oz	7–9
Cheese spread	1 oz	6–9
Colby	1 oz	9

		g Fat
Cottage, creamed, 4%	½ C	5
Cottage, with fruit	½ C	5
Cottage, dry curd	½ C	1
Cottage, 2%	½ C	4
Cottage, 1%	½ C	1
Cream	1 oz	10
Edam	1 oz	8
Feta	1 oz	6
Gouda	1 oz	8
Mozzarella	1 oz	7
Mozzarella, part skim	1 oz	5
Muenster	1 oz	9
Parmesan, grated	1 Tbsp	2
Provolone	1 oz	8
Ricotta, whole	½ C	16
Ricotta, part skim	½ C	10
Swiss	1 oz	8

Cream

light	1 Tbsp	3
light whipping	1 Tbsp	5
heavy whipping	1 Tbsp	6
whipped, pressurized	1 Tbsp	tr
sour	1 Tbsp	3
half and half	1 Tbsp	2
frozen whipped topping	1 Tbsp	1

Ice Cream

Vanilla

10% fat	1 C	14
16% fat	1 C	24

		g Fat
soft serve	1 C	23
Chocolate	1 C	16
Creamsicle	1 each	3
Drumstick	1 each	10
Fudgsicle	1 each	tr
Ice cream sandwich	1 each	6
Ice milk, all flavors	½ C	3
Ices, all flavors	1 C	tr
Popsicle	1 each	tr
Sherbet, all fruit flavors	½ C	0–2

Yogurt

coffee/vanilla, low-fat	1 C	3
fruited, low-fat	1 C	3
plain, regular	1 C	7
low-fat	1 C	4
skim	1 C	tr
frozen, soft serve, fruit flavor	1 C	2
chocolate	1 C	3
vanilla	1 C	2

DESSERTS AND SWEETS

		g Fat

Candy

Baby Ruth	1 oz	6
Butterfinger	1 oz	6
Caramels	1 each	1
Milk chocolate	1 oz	9
with almonds	1 oz	10

		g Fat
M & M's	1.7-oz pkg	10
Mr. Goodbar	1.65 oz bar	17
Hard or jellied candy	1 oz	0
Licorice	1 oz	tr
Snickers	2-oz bar	13
3 Musketeers	2.1-oz bar	8
Cheesecake	$\frac{1}{8}$	16
Cupcakes, Hostess	2	6
Ding Dongs/Big Wheels, Hostess	2	9
Ho Ho's, Hostess	1 each	6
Sno Balls, Hostess	1 each	4
Suzy Q's, Hostess	1 each	9
Twinkies, Hostess	1 each	5
Doughnut, plain	1 each	6–7
with icing	1 each	8
Gelatin, all flavors	$\frac{1}{2}$ C	tr
with 1 Tbsp whipped cream	$\frac{1}{2}$ C	1
Eclair with chocolate icing and custard filling	1 each	15
Pastry crust, frozen	$\frac{1}{8}$ pie	16
Pie, frozen		
Apple	$\frac{1}{8}$ pie	17
Banana cream	$\frac{1}{8}$ pie	12
Cherry	$\frac{1}{8}$ pie	16
Chocolate cream	$\frac{1}{8}$ pie	13
Coconut cream	$\frac{1}{8}$ pie	14
Coconut custard	$\frac{1}{8}$ pie	15
Custard	$\frac{1}{8}$ pie	9

		g Fat
Lemon cream	⅛ pie	12
Lemon meringue	⅛ pie	10
Pecan	⅛ pie	23
Pumpkin custard	⅛ pie	11
Pie fillings, canned		
Apple	⅛ pie	0
Banana cream	⅛ pie	2
Cherry	⅛ pie	0
Chocolate	⅛ pie	2
Coconut cream	⅛ pie	3
Lemon meringue	⅛ pie	1.5
Pumpkin	⅛ pie	0
Vanilla cream	⅛ pie	3
Snack pie		
Apple, Hostess	1 pie	20
Blueberry, Hostess	1 pie	20
Cherry, Hostess	1 pie	20
Lemon, Hostess	1 pie	22
Peach, Hostess	1 pie	20
Pudding		
Banana cream	½ C	4
Butter pecan	½ C	5
Butterscotch	½ C	4
low cal	½ C	tr
Chocolate	½ C	5
Rice	½ C	4
Tapioca	½ C	4
Vanilla		
(with whole milk)	½ C	4
(with skim milk)	½ C	tr
Pudding Pops, Jell-O	1 each	2

EGGS

		g Fat
Fresh, whole	1 egg	6
Omelet, plain	1 egg	7
Egg yolk	1 egg	6
Egg white	1 egg	tr
Egg substitute, liquid	1½ oz	2

FAST FOOD

g Fat

Burger King

		g Fat
BK Broiler Chicken Sandwich		
with sauce	as served	18
without sauce	as served	8
Burger Buddies	as served	17
Chicken Tenders	as served	13
Chicken Sandwich (fried)	as served	40
Cheeseburger	as served	15
Chef Salad (without dressing)	as served	9
Chunky Chicken Salad, without dressing	as served	4
Croissan'wich	as served	40
Double Whopper with cheese	as served	61
French fries	as served	13
Hamburger	as served	11
Hamburger Deluxe	as served	19
Scrambled Egg Platter with sausage	as served	53

		g Fat
Whopper	as served	38
Whopper,		
with cheese	as served	45
Whopper Jr.	as served	17
Hardee's		
Bacon Cheese-		
burger	as served	39
Big Country Breakfast		
with ham	as served	38
with sausage	as served	57
Big Deluxe Burger ...	as served	30
Chef Salad		
(without dressing)	as served	15
Chicken 'N' Pasta		
Salad	as served	3
Chicken Stix	6 pieces	9
Fisherman's Fillet	as served	24
Grilled Chicken		
Sandwich	as served	9
Hamburger	as served	10
Mushroom 'N' Swiss		
Burger	as served	27
The Lean 1		
Hamburger	as served	18
Three pancakes	as served	2
with sausage	as served	16
Kentucky Fried Chicken		
Original Recipe, side		
or center breast	1 (3.5 oz)	15
drumstick	1 (2 oz)	9

		g Fat
Mashed potatoes w/gravy	as served	1
Corn on the cob	as served	3
Cole slaw	as served	6
Baked beans	as served	1

McDonald's

Big Mac	as served	26
Biscuit with sausage & egg	as served	33
Chicken McNuggets	6 pieces	17
Chunky Chicken Salad	as served	4
Egg McMuffin	as served	12
Fillet-O-Fish	as served	26
without tartar sauce	as served	10
French fries, regular	as served	12
Hamburger	as served	9
Hotcakes with margarine and syrup	as served	9
McLean Deluxe	as served	10
Quarter Pounder with cheese	as served	28
Sausage McMuffin	as served	11
with egg	as served	25

Pizza Hut

Thin 'N Crispy Cheese, 10″	3 slices	15
Thin 'N Chewy Cheese, 10″	3 slices	14

Taco Bell

Bean Burrito	as served	11

		g Fat
Burrito Supreme	as served	19
Mexican Pizza	as served	37
Nachos BellGrande	as served	35
Nachos Supreme	as served	27
Soft Taco	as served	12
Soft Taco Supreme	as served	16
Taco	as served	11
Taco BellGrande	as served	23
Taco Salad	as served	61
Tostada with red sauce	as served	11
Wendy's		
Big Classic Hamburger	as served	33
Chili, large	as served	12
Crispy Chicken Nuggets	as served	20
Fish Fillet Sandwich	as served	25
Garden Spot Salad Bar		
cole slaw	$\frac{1}{4}$ C	5
pasta salad	$\frac{1}{4}$ C	6
cottage cheese	$\frac{1}{2}$ C	4
breadsticks	4	2
Grilled Chicken Fillet, no sauce	as served	3
Hamburger	as served	16
Hot Stuffed Baked Potato		
chili & cheese	as served	18
sour cream & chive	as served	23

	g Fat
Jr. Hamburger .... as served	9
Jr. Swiss Deluxe ...... as served	18
Plain baked potato ... as served	tr

FATS AND OILS

Remember, the harder the fat, the more saturated (artery-clogging) it is!!

		g Fat
Bacon fat	1 Tbsp	14
Beef, pork, or chicken fat	1 Tbsp	13
Butter	1 pat	4
	1 Tbsp	14
Crisco shortening	1 Tbsp	12
Margarine, stick or tub ...	1 pat	4
	1 Tbsp	11
Any vegetable oil	1 Tbsp	14
No-stick spray	2-second spray	tr
Salad dressing, bottled		
Blue cheese, regular ...	1 Tbsp	6–8
low cal	1 Tbsp	1–4
French, regular	1 Tbsp	5–6
low cal	1 Tbsp	2
Italian, regular	1 Tbsp	7–8
low cal	1 Tbsp	3
Russian, regular	1 Tbsp	5
low cal	1 Tbsp	1
Thousand Island	1 Tbsp	5–6
low cal	1 Tbsp	3
Mayonnaise	1 Tbsp	11
Imitation	1 Tbsp	3
Sandwich spread	1 Tbsp	5

FISH AND SHELLFISH

		g Fat
Bass, sea, broiled	3½ oz	13
Bluefish, broiled	3½ oz	6
Caviar	1 Tbsp	2
Cod, broiled/baked	3½ oz	5
Fishsticks	5	14
Haddock, broiled/baked	3½ oz	7
Halibut, broiled/baked	3½ oz	9
Herring, kippered	3½ oz	13
Mackerel, canned	4 oz	12
Ocean perch, fried	3½ oz	13
Salmon, coho, broiled/baked	3½ oz	7
sockeye, canned	⅖ C	9
Sardines, in oil	8	24
in tomato sauce	8	17
Smelt, canned	4–5	14
Sole, broiled/baked	3½ oz	1
Swordfish, broiled/baked	3½ oz	6
Trout, broiled/baked	3½ oz	11
Tuna, fresh, raw, yellowfin	4 oz	1
canned, in oil	2 oz	12
canned, in water	2 oz	1
in water, salad w/mayo	½ C	11
Whitefish, smoked	3½ oz	7
Shellfish:		
Abalone, raw	4 oz	tr

		g Fat
Clams, raw	4 lg	2
Crab, steamed	4 oz	2
Lobster, boiled/ broiled w/butter	$^3/_4$ lb	25
Oyster, raw	5–8 med	3
Scallops, steamed	$3^1/_2$ oz	1
Shrimp, breaded/fried	$3^1/_2$ oz	11
Squid (calamari), raw	$3^1/_2$ oz	1

FRUITS AND BERRIES

Most fruits and berries contain only TRACE amounts of fat!!! The exceptions include the following:

		g Fat
Avocado, raw	1 med	30
Cherimoya, raw	1 med	2
Coconut, dried, shredded	$^1/_3$ C	9
Figs, dried	10	2
Guava, strawberry, raw	1 C	2
Jujube, raw	$3^1/_2$ oz	1
Lychees, dried	$3^1/_2$ oz	1
Sapodilla, raw	1 med	2
Sapotes, raw	1 med	1

GRAVIES AND SAUCES

		g Fat
BBQ Sauce	1 Tbsp	tr
Béarnaise, dehydrated	9-oz pkt	2
Curry, dry	1.2-oz pkt	8

		g Fat
Hollandaise, mix, prepared w/ water...	3 Tbsp	4
Homemade drippings with flour	1/4 C	12
Homestyle gravy, mix, prepared w/ water...	1/4 C	1
Ketchup	1 Tbsp	tr
Mushroom gravy, canned	2 oz	1
Mustard, brown or yellow	1 Tbsp	tr
Steak sauce	1 Tbsp	tr
Stroganoff, mix	1.2-oz pkt	tr
Sweet-n-Sour	1 Tbsp	tr
Tartar sauce	1 Tbsp	8
Teriyaki, bottled	1 Tbsp	tr
White sauce, mix	1-oz pkt	11
Worcestershire	1 Tbsp	0

LIQUORS

Alcohol has lots of calories but no fat unless mixed with cream, milk, or whipped cream.

MEAT AND POULTRY

*Remember, the leaner the meat, the lower the fat content.
*Lean cuts of meat include: Fillet, Flank, Rump Round, Sirloin, Tenderloin.
*White meat poultry is leaner than dark meat poultry.
*Most poultry fat is located in and around the skin.

Beef

Brisket,		
lean trimmed	4 oz	15
Chipped	3 oz	5
creamed	½ C	13
Corned hash,		
canned	3½ oz	11
Flank, lean, braised,		
trimmed	4 oz	16
Ground, broiled,		
extra lean	4 oz	19
lean		23
regular		30
Porterhouse, broiled,		
trimmed	4 oz	12
Ribs, whole,		
roasted	6–12 ribs	37
Round bottom, braised,		
trimmed	4 oz	11
top, fried, trimmed	4 oz	10
Sirloin, broiled,		
trimmed	4 oz	10
T-bone steak, broiled,		
trimmed	4 oz	12
Tenderloin, broiled,		
trimmed	4 oz	8

Organ meats

Brains, beef, raw	4 oz	11
Heart, beef, braised	4 oz	6
Kidney, beef,		
braised	4 oz	4

Liver, beef,
pan-fried .... 3½ oz 11

Sweetbread (thymus),
beef, braised .... 3½ oz 23

Tongue, beef, smoked 3½ oz 29

Poultry

Broilers/fryers, white meat
with skin, fried ...... 3½ oz 12
without skin, fried ... 3½ oz 6
with skin, roasted .. 3½ oz 11
without skin,
roasted .... 3½ oz 5

Broilers/fryers, dark meat
with skin, fried .. ... 3½ oz 17
without skin, fried ... 3½ oz 12
with skin, roasted .... 3½ oz 16
without skin,
roasted .... 3½ oz 10

Chicken giblets,
fried .... 3½ oz 14

Duck, roasted,
with skin .... 3½ oz 28
without skin .... 3½ oz 11

Goose, roasted,
with skin .... 3½ oz 22
without skin .... 3½ oz 13

Turkey, white meat, roasted,
with skin .... 3½ oz 8
without skin .... 3½ oz 3

Turkey, dark meat, roasted,
with skin .... 3½ oz 12

		g Fat
without skin	3½ oz	7
Turkey, ground,		
cooked	3½ oz	14
Lamb		
Blade chop, lean with fat,		
broiled	3½ oz	26
Leg of, lean with fat,		
roasted	3½ oz	15
Loin chop, lean with fat,		
broiled	3½ oz	23
Rib chop, lean with fat,		
broiled	3½ oz	37
Pork		
Bacon, broiled/fried		
crisp	3 oz	9
Bacon, Canadian,		
broiled/fried	1 slice	4
Bacon Bits	1 Tbsp	2
Blade, lean with fat,		
broiled	3½ oz	29
Ham, smoked,		
cooked	3½ oz	11
Loin chop, lean with fat,		
broiled	3½ oz	26
Picnic shoulder, lean with fat,		
braised	3½ oz	24
Spareribs, lean with fat,		
roasted	3 med	18
Sausages and luncheon meats		
Beerwurst (beef)	1 slice	6
Blood sausage	1 slice	9

		g Fat
Bologna (beef or pork)	1 slice	7
Bratwurst (pork)	1 link	22
Brotwurst (pork or beef)	1 link	20
Chicken roll (white meat)	1 slice	2
Frankfurter (beef or pork)	1 link	13
(chicken)	1 link	9
(turkey)	1 link	8
Ham, chopped, canned	1 slice	4
Ham, sliced (5% fat)	1 slice	1
(11% fat)	1 slice	3
Ham and cheese loaf	1 slice	6
Italian sausage (pork)	1 link	17
Kielbasa (pork or beef)	1 slice	7
Knockwurst (pork or beef)	1 link	19
Liverwurst (pork)	1 slice	5
Mortadella (beef and pork)	1 slice	4
Olive loaf (pork)	1 slice	5
Pâté, goose liver	1 oz	12
Pickle and pimento loaf (pork)	1 slice	6

		g Fat
Polish sausage (pork)	1 oz	8
Pork sausage, link	1 link	22
patty	1 patty	13
Salami (beef or pork)	1 slice	5
Turkey breast	1 slice	tr
Turkey pastrami	1 slice	2
Turkey roll (white and dark meat)	1 slice	2
(white meat only)	1 slice	2
Vienna sausage, canned (beef or pork)	1 link	4

NUTS AND SEEDS

		g Fat
Almonds, dry-roasted	1 oz	15
Brazil nuts, shelled	6 lg	19
Cashews, dry-roasted	1 oz	13
Mixed nuts, dry-roasted	1 oz	15
Peanuts, dry-roasted	1 oz	14
Peanut butter	2 Tbsp	17
Pecans, dry-roasted	1 oz	18
Pumpkin seeds, dry, whole	4 oz	39
Sesame seeds, whole	1 Tbsp	4
Sunflower seeds, whole	1 oz	16
Walnuts, shelled	1 oz	18

SOUPS AND BROTHS

		g Fat
Asparagus, cream of, canned		

		g Fat
made w/milk	1 C	8
made w/water	1 C	4
Bean w/bacon	1 C	6
Bean w/ franks	1 C	7
Bean w/ ham	1 C	9
Beef broth/bouillon	1 C	tr
Beef, chunky	1 C	5
Beef mushroom	1 C	3
Beef noodle	1 C	3
Celery, cream of		
made w/milk	1 C	10
made w/water	1 C	6
Cheese, condensed		
made w/milk	1 C	15
made w/water	1 C	11
Chicken and		
dumpling	1 C	6
Chicken broth	1 C	1
Chicken, chunky	1 C	7
Chicken, cream of		
made w/milk	1 C	12
made w/water	1 C	7
Chicken gumbo	1 C	1
Chicken mushroom	1 C	9
Chicken noodle	1 C	3
Chicken rice	1 C	2
Chicken vegetable	1 C	3
Clam chowder		
Manhattan style	1 C	3
New England style		
made w/milk	1 C	7

		g Fat
made w/water	1 C	3
Lentil w/ham	1 C	3
Minestrone, chunky	1 C	3
Mushroom, cream of		
made w/milk	1 C	14
made w/water	1 C	9
Onion, cream of		
made w/milk	1 C	9
made w/water	1 C	5
Split pea w/ham	1 C	4
Scotch broth	1 C	3
Tomato		
made w/milk	1 C	6
made w/water	1 C	2
Turkey noodle	1 C	2
Turkey vegetable	1 C	3
Vegetable beef	1 C	2
Vegetable,		
vegetarian	1 C	2
Wonton	1 C	2
Dehydrated		
Beef broth	1 cube	tr
Chicken broth	1 cube	1
Onion soup mix	1 pkt	1

SUGARS

		g Fat
Sugar, brown, powdered, or white	1 Tbsp	0

Syrups:

		g Fat
Corn	1 Tbsp	0
Maple	1 Tbsp	0
Log Cabin, buttered	1 Tbsp	tr

VEGETABLES

Most vegetables contain only TRACE amounts of fat!!! Watch out for cream, butter, or cheese sauces, mayonnaise, hollandaise sauce, and almondine dishes. These ingredients can add anywhere from 3 to 12 grams of fat per serving. Be sure to read the labels of all canned and frozen vegetables. The exceptions to this rule include the following:

		g Fat
Beans, BBQ, canned	1 C	4
brown sugar	1 C	6
chili, Mexican style	1 C	3
homestyle	1 C	4
and pork	1 C	4
Chiles, red, raw	3½ oz	3
dried	1¾ oz	5
Corn on the cob	4-inch ear	1
Garbanzo beans, canned	3½ oz	2
Soybean curd (tofu)	½ oz	4
Soybean sprouts	1 C	1
Soybeans immature, cooked, canned	⅔ C	5
mature, cooked	½ C	6

fermented (miso)	3½ oz	5
(natto)	3½ oz	7
Tomato paste, canned	1 C	1
Tomato puree, canned	29-oz can	2
Turnip greens, canned, chopped	1 C	1
Yellow eye beans, baked, canned	⅞ C	7

Seven Low-Fat, High-Taste Menus

DAY 1

Breakfast
½ C orange juice
¾ C bran flakes cereal
1 C 1% or skim milk
1 small banana
coffee or tea

Lunch
Turkey sandwich
    2 oz turkey breast
    1 Tbsp diet mayonnaise
    lettuce, tomato
    2 slices whole wheat or rye bread
1 apple
1 C fruit juice and/or diet soft drink

Dinner

3–4 oz chicken breast, skinned, baked with BBQ
    sauce
Corn on the cob with 1 tsp tub margarine
Green beans with 1 tsp tub margarine
Fresh vegetable salad with wine vinegar and basil
1 crusty roll with 1 tsp tub margarine
1 C fresh fruit salad

Snack

1 C 1% or skim milk
3–4 ginger snaps

1700 calories
52 g fat (3½ Tbsp)
27% fat
4% saturated fat
127 mg cholesterol

DAY 2

Breakfast

½ grapefruit
½ C hot oatmeal with 1–2 Tbsp raisins and cinna-
    mon to taste
1 C 1% or skim milk
coffee or tea

Lunch

Roast beef sandwich
    2 oz lean roast beef
    1 Tbsp diet mayonnaise
    lettuce, tomato

1 hard roll
1 orange
1 C 1% or skim milk or fruit juice

Dinner
Pasta Primavera
    1 C pasta (any variety)
    steamed mixed vegetables
    tomato sauce
    sprinkled with 2 oz part skim mozzarella and
        Parmesan cheese
Fresh vegetable salad with 1 tsp olive oil and wine
      vinegar
$1/4$ canteloupe or honeydew

Snack
$1/2$ C ice milk with $1/4$ C fresh blueberries or rasp-
    berries

1400 calories
43 g fat (2$1/2$ Tbsp)
27% fat
7% saturated fat
87 mg cholesterol

DAY 3

Breakfast
$1/2$ C fruit juice
Scrambled eggs
    with $1/4$ C egg substitute and
    $1/4$ C 1% or skim milk in nonstick pan

2 slices whole wheat toast with 2 tsp jam
coffee or tea

Lunch
Tuna Boat
   2 oz water-pack tuna
   1 Tbsp diet mayonnaise
   celery, onion and spices to taste
1 whole tomato (stuffed with tuna)
$1/2$ bagel with 1 tsp tub margarine
1 C 1% or skim milk

Dinner
3–4 oz broiled orange roughy or cod in lemon
   juice, sprinkled with paprika
Steamed broccoli
Large baked potato with 1 tsp tub margarine and
   1 Tbsp plain nonfat yogurt
Fresh vegetable salad with 2 Tbsp fat-free salad
   dressing
1 C fresh melon
Diet soft drink

Snack
$1/2$ C fruit sorbet and $3/4$ C fresh strawberries

1500 calories
48 g fat (3 Tbsp)
29% fat
5% saturated fat
144 mg cholesterol

DAY 4

Breakfast

$\frac{1}{4}$ fresh melon

1 whole wheat English muffin with 1 oz melted
   part skim mozzarella

1 C 1% or skim milk

coffee or tea

Lunch

1 C soup (pasta and bean, lentil, minestrone, or
   vegetarian split pea)

Chef's salad

   assorted fresh vegetables

   1 oz turkey breast strips

   1 oz. ham strips

   1 Tbsp low-fat salad dressing

Flavored seltzer water

Dinner

3–4 oz lean beef (flank, round, sirloin or tenderloin), broiled with sautéed mushrooms in 1
   tsp olive oil

Medium sweet potato, baked with 1 tsp tub margarine and a dash of nutmeg and cinnamon

Steamed zucchini and pearl onions

1 clover leaf roll with 1 tsp tub margarine

1 poached pear

Snack

1 C 1% or skim milk

1 oz Entenmann's fat-free dessert

1450 calories
48 g fat (3 Tbsp)
29% fat
6% saturated fat
142 mg cholesterol

DAY 5

Breakfast
$\frac{1}{2}$ C fruit juice
1 C low-fat fruited yogurt
1 whole wheat English muffin with 1 tsp tub margarine and 1 tsp jam
coffee or tea

Lunch
Grilled cheese sandwich
  2 oz part skim mozzarella or other low-fat cheese
  2 slices whole wheat bread with 1 tsp tub margarine in a nonstick pan
1 C tomato soup sprinkled with grated Parmesan cheese
1 C 1% or skim milk

Dinner
$\frac{1}{2}$ lb Cornish hen glazed with orange marmalade
Fresh steamed spinach with water chestnuts
$\frac{1}{2}$ C brown and wild rice with 1 tsp tub margarine
1 hard crusty roll with 1 tsp tub margarine
$\frac{1}{2}$ C green and red grapes
Flavored seltzer water

Snack
Fruit smoothie, blended (1 small frozen banana cut
into chunks; 1 C 1% or skim milk; ice cubes)

1800 calories
61 g fat (4 Tbsp)
30% fat
6% saturated fat
134 mg cholesterol

DAY 6

Breakfast
$\frac{1}{2}$ grapefruit
$\frac{1}{2}$ C hot oat bran cereal with fresh blueberries
1 C 1% or skim milk
coffee or tea

Lunch
Ham sandwich
    2 slices ham
    lettuce, tomato
    mustard or 1 Tbsp fat-free mayonnaise
    2 slices whole grain bread
1 fresh nectarine or peach
1 C 1% or skim milk

Dinner
3–4 oz grilled salmon fillet with spices to taste
$\frac{1}{2}$ C pasta with 1 tsp tub margarine and grated
    Parmesan cheese
Fresh vegetable salad with any variety fat-free
    dressing

$^1/_2$ C fresh fruit salad

Snack
1 C 1% or skim milk
2 Fig Newtons

1450 calories
48 g fat (3 Tbsp)
26% fat
6% saturated fat
142 mg cholesterol

DAY 7

Breakfast
$^1/_4$ melon
2 whole grain waffles
2 Tbsp maple syrup
1 C 1% or skim milk
coffee or tea

Lunch
Curry chicken salad sandwich
    2 oz white meat chicken
    1 Tbsp diet mayonnaise
    dash curry
    $^1/_2$ apple, chunked
    celery
    2 Tbsp walnut pieces
    1 large pita pocket, stuffed
2 tangerines
1 C fruit juice

Dinner

3–4 oz pork or veal medallions with apricot pre-
serves

1 C brown rice combined with steamed broccoli
florets with 1 tsp tub margarine

Fresh vegetable salad with 1 tsp olive oil and wine
vinegar

$\frac{1}{2}$ C unsweetened applesauce

$\frac{1}{2}$ C fruit sorbet

Snack

$\frac{1}{2}$ bagel with 1 Tbsp low-fat cream cheese

1 C 1% or skim milk

2000 calories

65 g fat (4$\frac{1}{2}$ Tbsp)

29% fat

4% saturated fat

130 mg cholesterol

SELECTED REFERENCES

1. USDA Handbook No. 8 Series: *Composition of Foods.*

2. Bowes and Church's *Food Values of Portions Commonly Used.* Revised by Jean A. T. Pennington, Ph.D., R.D., and Helen Nichols Church, B.S., J. B. Lippincott Co., Philadelphia, 1985.

3. Tufts University Diet & Nutrition Letter, published by Tufts University, Boston, Mass., 1987–91. Editor: Stanley N. Gershoff, Ph.D., Dean, School of Nutrition.

4. Nutrition Action Health Letter, published by Center for Science in the Public Interest, Washington, D.C., 1989–91. Executive Editor: Michael Jacobson, Ph.D.

SUSAN KAGEN PODELL is a clinical nutritionist and registered dietitian who has worked at both the New York University Medical Center and Boston's Massachusetts General Hospital, and in private practice. She is the author of *The Vest Pocket Cholesterol Counter.* She lives in Columbus, Ohio.